LIVING WITH AMYLOIDOSIS: A DIET COOKBOOK FOR BEGINNERS

Your Roadmap to Symptom Relief, Improved Kidney Function, and Protecting Your Immune System

Daria Cross, RD

COPYRIGHT PAGE

The information in this book is not intended, under any circumstances, to replace or serve as a substitute for professional medical advice, diagnosis, or treatment. Any individual seeking advice regarding a medical condition or seeking treatment options should always consult with a qualified healthcare provider or physician. The author and publisher explicitly disclaim any responsibility for adverse effects or consequences arising from the utilization of the recipes or information presented in this cookbook.

Table of Contents

PART 1: INTRODUCTION TO AMYLOIDOSIS

Amyloidosis is a rare disorder that happens when proteins in your body change or mutate, becoming twisted clumps of misshapen proteins that gather on your organs and tissues. Amyloidosis can be widespread (systemic) or localized to one area. Systemic is the most common form of amyloidosis, affecting organs and multiple tissues. In some instances, systemic amyloidosis may cause life-threatening organ damage. Localized amyloidosis only affects one organ or part of your body. There are several types of amyloidosis. Some types affect specific organs such as your heart, kidneys, liver and nerves. Other types spread throughout your body. Healthcare providers can't cure amyloidosis, but they can slow its progress and ease symptoms.

Overview of Amyloidosis

Healthcare providers call amyloidosis a "protein misfolding disorder." Your proteins are long molecules that stretch out in long chains. They're multitaskers that do everything from providing energy, balancing fluids and helping with immunity to providing structure, carrying material and regulating your body's processes. Normally, proteins leave your bloodstream once they finish their assigned tasks. In protein misfolding disorder, proteins take on abnormal shapes that get deposited in many organs, can't be removed and your body can't use.

These abnormal proteins navigate your bloodstream and find their way to healthy organs. They tend to clump together, making amyloid deposits (or fibrils) that may build up on different organs or in different places throughout your body.

Systemic amyloidosis may affect just about any organ, heart, kidneys, liver, GI tract, joints, skin and blood vessels. Sometimes, the amyloid deposits build up so much that they can cause organ failure. Think of debris floating down a river that snags on a rock or tree limb. Over time, more and more debris catches in the snag, forcing the river to flow around the large snag. Just like debris caught on a snag, amyloid deposits accumulate within organs, eventually affecting organ structure and tissue function. Sometimes, amyloid deposits caused by systemic amyloidosis can literally take over healthy organs, replacing the organs with amyloid deposits.

Localized amyloidosis typically affects your skin, bladder and airways.

Causes and Types of Amyloidosis

Amyloidosis occurs when the body produces amyloid proteins. The reason amyloids develop may vary, depending on the type of amyloidosis present.

There are many different types of amyloidosis. Some types are hereditary. Others are caused by outside factors, such as inflammatory diseases or long-term dialysis. Many types affect multiple organs. Others affect only one part of the body.

Types of amyloidosis include:

AL amyloidosis (immunoglobulin light chain amyloidosis): This is the most common type of amyloidosis in developed countries. AL amyloidosis is also called primary amyloidosis. It usually affects the heart, kidneys, liver and nerves.

AA amyloidosis: This type is also known as secondary amyloidosis. It's usually triggered by an inflammatory disease, such as rheumatoid arthritis. It most commonly affects the kidneys, liver and spleen.

Hereditary amyloidosis (familial amyloidosis): This inherited disorder often affects the nerves, heart and kidneys. It most commonly happens when a protein made by your liver is abnormal. This protein is called transthyretin (TTR).

Wild-type amyloidosis: This variety has also been called senile systemic amyloidosis. It occurs when the TTR protein made by the liver is normal but produces amyloid for unknown reasons. Wild-type amyloidosis tends to affect men over age 70 and often targets the heart. It can also cause carpal tunnel syndrome.

Localized amyloidosis: This type of amyloidosis often has a better prognosis than the varieties that affect multiple organ systems. Typical sites for localized amyloidosis include the bladder, skin, throat or lungs. Correct diagnosis is important so that treatments that affect the entire body can be avoided.

Risk Factors

Although anyone can develop amyloidosis, certain factors increase a person's risk of the disease. These include:

Age: Amyloidosis can develop in young adults, but the most common form of amyloidosis occurs more often between 50 and 80 years of age.

Family history: There is a genetic form of amyloidosis, so having a close blood relative, such as a parent, with the condition may increase a person's risk.

Sex: Approximately two-thirds of people with AL amyloidosis are male.

Dialysis: People who undergo long-term dialysis to treat kidney disease are at an increased risk of developing a specific form of amyloidosis.

History of inflammatory disease: Some conditions, such as arthritis or inflammatory bowel disease, can trigger AA amyloidosis. According to the National Organization for Rare Diseases, about 50% of people with AA amyloidosis have rheumatoid arthritis.

Diagnosis of Amyloidosis

The symptoms of amyloidosis can mimic other diseases. For example, symptoms that affect kidney function may lead to a misdiagnosis of other renal conditions.

Since amyloidosis is a rare disease, it may take some time for doctors to make a diagnosis. Correctly diagnosing amyloidosis is essential to target the most effective treatment.

Diagnostic testing for amyloidosis may include:

Tissue biopsy: A tissue biopsy involves removing a small sample of tissue to check for amyloid deposits. A doctor typically takes a sample from a fat pad under the skin in the abdomen or from an organ.

Bone marrow biopsy: Removal of bone marrow involves checking for the presence of amyloid deposits. Doctors will usually take the bone marrow from the pelvic bone.

Blood and urine tests: Various urine and blood tests can help determine which organs are involved. For example, urine tests may indicate kidney damage, whereas blood tests may measure problems with the heart.

Symptoms of Amyloidosis

The buildup of amyloid proteins interferes with the normal functions of the organs. Symptoms can vary, however, depending on which organs amyloidosis affects.

Common symptoms may include:

weakness

unexplained weight loss

edema, or swelling

nausea

chest pain

dizziness

abnormal heart rhythm

bruising around the eyes

hoarseness

Occasionally, amyloid deposits may buildup on a specific organ without widespread development in other areas. For example, amyloids may deposit on the skin, bladder, or larynx.

It is more common, however, for amyloidosis to affect more than one organ.

Treatment Strategies

There is currently no cure for amyloidosis, but the condition is treatable.

Treatment involves slowing the progression of the disease, decreasing symptoms, and improving a person's quality of life.

Treatment depends on the severity of symptoms and the type of amyloidosis.

Possible therapies to decrease amyloid protein development include:

Chemotherapy

Chemotherapy is the use of various drugs to kill the abnormal blood cells that help form amyloids.

Medications for myeloma, which is cancer of the plasma cells, can sometimes be an option.

A doctor may recommend the following chemotherapy drugs:

melphalan

bendamustine

cyclophosphamide

bortezomib

The type of chemotherapy a person receives will depend on the extent of their symptoms, their age, and which organs symptoms affect.

Other medications

Immunomodulatory drugs are oral medications that modify the action of the immune system. Approved medications include:

thalidomide

lenalidomide

pomalidomide

Monoclonal antibodies are proteins that act like the body's natural immune system. Daratumumab (in combination with other agents) was the first Food and Drug Administration (FDA)-approved monoclonal antibody for newly diagnosed AL amyloidosis. It may be given intravenously or by injection under the skin.

Transthyretin stabilization agents are specifically indicated for ATTR cardiac amyloidosis. Tafamidis has been shown to decrease death and cardiovascular hospitalizations.

Stem cell transplant

In some instances, a doctor may recommend stem cell transplantation after chemotherapy.

After destroying the abnormal cells that produce amyloids with chemotherapy, stem cell transplants can help develop healthy bone marrow.

Receiving a stem cell transplantation is a complex process, and not every person with amyloidosis qualifies.

Controlling underlying diseases

Treatment for people with AA amyloidosis often includes managing underlying issues that lead to the buildup of amyloid.

Once a person treats the underlying condition, such as rheumatoid arthritis, they may experience fewer symptoms of amyloidosis.

Supportive treatment

A person may also need to treat complications of the disease or make changes in their diet or lifestyle to make managing the disease easier.

Supportive treatment can include a wide variety of medications and therapies, including:

medications to control heart failure

blood pressure medications

dialysis to treat kidney damage

nutritional support and guidance for those with digestive issues

PART 2: IMPORTANCE OF DIET IN MANAGING AMYLOIDOSIS

Digestive problems can be common in people with amyloidosis. The reason for these problems is the abnormal accumulation of proteins in their gastrointestinal tract. They are caused by a number of factors including inflammation of the gastrointestinal tract, impaired intestinal motility or malabsorption of nutrients. Commonly described symptoms include abdominal pain, nausea, vomiting, constipation or diarrhoea. These symptoms can be very debilitating and sometimes prevent patients from leaving their homes.

Consulting a doctor and dietician for advice and appropriate treatment can obviously help to manage the digestive symptoms associated with amyloidosis. However, the medicines prescribed by these health professionals do not provide real solutions to these problems. They only help to relieve patients. In addition to these medications, we offer advice on how to reduce digestive problems in people with these disorders.

Practical Advice for Managing Diet and Amyloidosis

It is essential that people with amyloidosis pay special attention to their diet. This could improve their quality of life and reduce the risk of complications related to their disease. Here are some nutrition tips:

Blond psyllium: this is a natural vegetable fibre that swells up to 40 times its volume in the presence of liquid. Mixed with water, it forms a gel that helps to regulate digestion. It is advised to take one tablespoon a day. It is very important to note that each dose must be taken at a distance from the medication (1 to 2 hours before or after taking the medication). Digestive improvements should appear after a few weeks.

Intermittent fasting: the two advantages of this practice are, on the one hand, that it feeds the digestive system and, on the other hand, its anti-inflammatory effect. There are many different forms of intermittent fasting. Jean-Christophe Fidalgo has opted for the one that seems simplest to him: the daily 14-hour fast. It is important to stay well hydrated during the fasting periods and to avoid sugary drinks. After a few days, you will feel comfortable with your digestive system.

Chrono-nutrition: its basic principle is to eat everything but not at any time. It is a question of grouping foods according to their speed of digestion: eat the foods that are heaviest to digest (fatty protein and slow sugar) at the beginning of the day. Avoid drinking during meals so as not to dissolve the digestive juices and slow down digestion.

Microbiota: it corresponds to the microorganisms (bacteria and fungi) that colonise our intestines. More and more studies show a link between the microbiota and various pathologies. It is important to enrich your microbiota through your diet: take lacto-fermented foods, eat yoghurts, fruit, vegetables and legumes rich in fibre, garlic and onions. In addition, you can also take a probiotic cure twice a year, preferably in autumn and spring, which will help improve your immune system.

PART 3: NUTRITIONAL CONSIDERATIONS FOR AMYLOIDOSIS PATIENTS

There is no specific amyloidosis diet plan or supplements that can prevent or treat amyloidosis. However, dietary modifications have helped some people feel better. A balanced diet that includes lean protein, healthy fats, fiber, and fruits and vegetables is recommended. In addition, if amyloidosis affects the heart or kidneys, a low-sodium diet may be recommended. It is also important to enrich your microbiota through your diet by taking lacto-fermented foods, eating yoghurts, fruit, vegetables and legumes rich in fibre, garlic and onions.

In summary, Opt for a diet rich in fruits, vegetables, whole grains, and lean proteins. Limit the intake of processed foods, sugary snacks, and saturated fats. Additionally, it is advisable to consult with a registered dietitian who can provide personalized dietary recommendations based on your specific needs.

Foods to Include

Carbohydrates: Opt for Whole Grains and Fiber for Optimal Health

Carbohydrates play a vital role in providing energy to your cells for various activities. They come in different forms:

• Sugars, or simple carbohydrates, serve as the foundational units for other carbohydrate types. Excess sugar not utilized by the body gets stored as fat.

• Starches are complex carbohydrates composed of long strings of simple sugars, taking longer to digest.

• Fiber, unlike other carbohydrates, remains undigested in the body, promoting digestive health, reducing constipation, regulating cholesterol and blood sugar levels, and lowering the risk of chronic diseases.

Consuming complex carbohydrates, such as starches and fiber, offers sustained energy levels and a feeling of fullness post-meal. Whole grains, like whole wheat bread or pasta, oatmeal, brown rice, popcorn, quinoa, and buckwheat, serve as excellent sources of complex carbohydrates, contributing significantly to overall well-being.

Additionally, vegetables and fruits prove to be excellent sources of healthy carbohydrates. Experts suggest filling half of your plate with non-starchy vegetables or fruits to optimize health benefits. These foods, along with legumes and whole grains, boast high fiber content, often lacking in many diets. To maximize nutritional intake, consuming fruits and vegetables with their skin intact and avoiding processed items is recommended. Beans, nuts, and seeds are also rich sources of dietary fiber.

Fats: Opt for Healthy Varieties and Avoid Saturated and Trans Fats

While fats often get a bad rap, they are essential for maintaining overall health. Fats provide energy, aid in vitamin absorption, regulate inflammation, and support skin, hair, and brain health.

However, not all fats are created equal. Saturated and trans fats, found in fatty meats, dairy products, and processed or fast food items, can elevate cholesterol levels and increase the risk of heart disease. On the contrary, monounsaturated and polyunsaturated fats, abundant in nuts, avocados, flax seeds, and fish, help in managing cholesterol levels and protecting against heart disease.

Opting for healthy oils like olive oil, corn oil, sunflower oil, safflower oil, and canola oil further promotes cardiovascular health.

Proteins: Strike a Balance with Lean Sources

Proteins are vital for maintaining healthy muscles, skin, and bones, as well as for hormone and enzyme production. It's crucial to include an adequate amount of protein in your daily diet for overall well-being.

While amyloidosis, a disease caused by abnormal protein buildup, may necessitate dietary adjustments for some individuals, lowering protein intake is generally unnecessary. The proteins obtained from food differ from the abnormal proteins associated with amyloidosis. However, individuals with amyloidosis who have kidney issues or are undergoing dialysis should be cautious with protein intake to avoid further kidney damage.

Opting for low-fat protein sources helps meet protein requirements while avoiding saturated fats. Lean meats, poultry, eggs, nuts, seeds, legumes, soy products, and seafood are excellent sources of healthy protein.

Vitamins and Minerals: Embrace a Colorful Diet

Vitamins and minerals are essential for cellular function and overall health. Consuming a variety of nutrient-rich foods from different food groups ensures adequate intake of essential vitamins and minerals.

Fruits and vegetables are rich sources of vitamins and minerals. Aim for a colorful diet as different-colored fruits and vegetables offer various nutrients. For instance:

• Red produce like tomatoes, grapefruit, and strawberries are rich in vitamin A, vitamin C, and antioxidants like lycopene.

• Orange and yellow fruits and vegetables such as carrots and bananas provide high levels of vitamin A, vitamin C, and potassium.

• Green produce like spinach and broccoli are abundant in vitamin K and potassium.

• Blue and purple fruits and veggies like blueberries, raisins, and eggplant offer antioxidants.

Consider supplementation if you suspect inadequate intake of vitamins and minerals, but consult your doctor before doing so, especially if you're undergoing treatment for amyloidosis, as certain supplements may interact with medication.

Hydration: Find the Right Balance

Staying hydrated is crucial for overall health, as water facilitates various bodily functions. However, individuals with conditions like amyloidosis need to be cautious about fluid intake, as excessive fluid retention can exacerbate heart or kidney issues associated with the condition. Consult your doctor for personalized guidance on fluid intake.

Amyloidogenic Foods to Limit or Avoid

Managing amyloidosis through diet involves being cautious of certain foods that can exacerbate symptoms and impact overall health. Here's a detailed look at foods to avoid:

1. **Saturated and Trans Fats**: It's wise to limit foods high in saturated and trans fats, commonly found in fatty meats, processed foods, fast food items, and certain dairy products. Opting for leaner protein sources and healthier fats like those found in nuts, seeds, and fish is advisable.

2. **High-Sodium Foods**: Excessive sodium intake can lead to fluid retention, worsening symptoms, particularly for those with heart or kidney complications. Processed foods, canned soups, salty snacks, and restaurant meals are often high in sodium. Choosing fresh, whole foods and flavoring

meals with herbs and spices instead of salt can help reduce sodium intake.

3. **Processed and Refined Carbohydrates**: Refined carbohydrates lack the fiber and nutrients found in whole grains and can cause spikes in blood sugar levels. Avoiding white bread, pastries, sugary snacks, and sugary beverages is recommended. Instead, focus on whole grains like whole wheat bread, brown rice, oats, and quinoa.

4. **High-Sugar Foods and Beverages**: Foods and beverages high in added sugars can contribute to weight gain and exacerbate insulin resistance. Sugary snacks, desserts, sugary drinks, and sweetened cereals should be limited or avoided. Opt for naturally sweet options like fruits, and use alternative sweeteners sparingly if needed.

5. **Alcohol:** Alcohol consumption can strain the liver and worsen symptoms, especially for those with liver involvement. Limiting or avoiding alcohol altogether is advisable. Instead, opt for hydrating beverages like water, herbal teas, or infused water with fruits and herbs.

6. **High-Protein Foods (for Certain Cases):** Individuals with kidney issues or undergoing dialysis may need to restrict protein intake to prevent further kidney damage. High-protein foods like fatty meats and processed meats should be consumed in moderation. Lean protein sources like poultry, fish, legumes, and tofu can help meet protein needs without overburdening the kidneys.

7. **Caffeine and Stimulants**: Stimulants like caffeine found in coffee, tea, energy drinks, and certain medications can increase heart rate and blood pressure, potentially worsening symptoms. Limiting caffeine intake or opting for decaffeinated beverages can help manage symptoms.

PART 4: RECIPES AND MEAL IDEAS FOR AMYLOIDOSIS DIET

TASTY, YUMMY RECIPES FOR BREAKFAST

Smoothie bowl

Ingredients

200g frozen mixed berries

1 ripe banana

75ml oat milk

1 tsp maple syrup

½ tbsp vanilla protein powder, vegan version if needed

To top

sliced kiwis, bananas and fresh berries

25g granola

1 tbsp mixed nuts and seeds

1 tbsp almond butter

Directions

STEP 1

Put the berries, banana, oat milk, maple syrup and protein powder in a powerful blender and blend until smooth. Add a splash more milk if needed, but remember it needs to be quite thick.

STEP 2

Spoon the smoothie into a bowl and dot over the fresh fruit, granola and mixed nuts and seeds. Drizzle over the almond butter to serve.

Healthy homemade granola

Ingredients

290g can pitted prunes in natural juice, drained

1 orange, zested and juiced

2 tbsp tahini

350g oats

25g flaked almonds

25g sunflower seeds

25g pumpkin seeds

2 x 400g pots fortified soya or plain bio yogurt

Directions

STEP 1

Heat the oven to 200C/180C fan/gas 6 and line a large baking tray with baking parchment. Put the prunes, orange zest and juice in a small bowl, add the tahini and mash it all together to make a paste. Tip the oats into a large bowl, then add the prune mixture and knead it all together using your hands, as though you're making a crumble topping, until all the oats are coated and sticky. Spread out on the prepared tray and bake for 20 mins, turning the oats every 5 mins to help them cook evenly and drive off as much steam as possible.

STEP 2

Remove from the oven and stir the almonds and seeds onto the tray, then cool quickly by tossing the mixture. Once completely cooled, the granola will keep for two weeks in an airtight container.

STEP 3

Measure 50g granola per serving and enjoy with 100g soya yogurt.

Breakfast peppers & chickpeas with tofu

Ingredients

1-2 tbsp olive oil

2 onions (320g), halved and thinly sliced

1 orange pepper, halved, deseeded and sliced

1 red chilli, deseeded and sliced

400g can chopped tomatoes

2 tbsp tomato purée

2 tsp vegetable bouillon powder

1 tsp dried oregano

1 tsp smoked paprika, plus extra for sprinkling

2 x 400g cans chickpeas

280g pack extra-firm tofu

240g soya yogurt

2 garlic cloves, finely grated

4 tbsp chopped parsley

Directions

STEP 1

Heat 1 tbsp oil in a large, deep frying pan over a medium heat. Tip in the onions, cover and cook for 5 mins. Remove the lid and stir the onions – they should have softened and started to brown in places. Stir in the pepper, chilli, chopped tomatoes, tomato purée, bouillon powder, oregano, paprika and chickpeas, along with the liquid from the cans. Cover and simmer for 15-20 mins until slightly thickened.

STEP 2

Meanwhile, slice half the tofu and fry in ½ tbsp oil over a medium heat until lightly golden. Combine the yogurt and garlic in a small bowl. Serve half the tomato and chickpea mixture with the tofu, half the yogurt and a scattering of parsley and extra paprika. Leave the leftovers to cool completely and chill the remaining chickpea mixture and yogurt for up to three days. Reheat the chickpea mixture in a small pan with a splash of water until piping hot, then fry the remaining tofu as above before serving.

Crispy hash browns

Ingredients

3 medium-sized potatoes (approx. 370g in total, unpeeled, left whole – Maris Pipers, King Edward and Desirée are all good choices)

50g butter, melted

4 tbsp sunflower oil

Directions

STEP 1

Cook the potatoes in a saucepan of boiling water for 10 mins then drain and set aside until cool enough to handle.

STEP 2

Coarsely grate the potatoes into a bowl discarding any skin that comes off in your hand as you grate. Season well with salt and pepper and pour over half the butter. Mix well then divide the mix into 8 and shape into patties or squares. The hash browns can be prepared a day ahead and chilled until ready to cook or frozen for up to a month.

STEP 3

To cook, heat the oil and the remaining butter in a frying pan until sizzling and gently fry the hash browns, in batches if needed, for 4-5 mins on each side until crisp and golden. Serve straight away or leave in a low oven to keep warm.

Mushroom hash with poached eggs

Ingredients

1 ½ tbsp avocado oil

2 large onions, halved and sliced

500g closed cup mushrooms, quartered

1 tbsp fresh thyme leaves, plus extra for sprinkling

500g fresh tomatoes, chopped

1 tsp smoked paprika

4 tsp omega seed mix (see tip)

4 large eggs

Directions

STEP 1

Heat the oil in a large non-stick frying pan and fry
the onions for a few mins. Cover the pan and leave
the onions to cook in their own steam for 5 mins
more.

STEP 2

Tip in the mushrooms with the thyme and cook,
stirring frequently, for 5 mins until softened. Add

the tomatoes and paprika, cover the pan and cook for 5 mins until pulpy. Stir through the seed mix.

STEP 3

If you're making this recipe as part of our two-person Summer Healthy Diet Plan, poach two of the eggs in lightly simmering water to your liking. Serve on top of half the hash with a sprinkling of fresh thyme and some black pepper. Chill the remaining hash to warm in a pan and eat with freshly poached eggs on another day. If you're serving four people, poach all four eggs, divide the hash between four plates, sprinkle with thyme and black pepper and serve with the eggs on top.

Spinach & Feta Scrambled Egg Pitas

Ingredients

1 tablespoon extra-virgin olive oil

1 (10 ounce) block frozen chopped spinach, thawed, drained and squeezed dry

Pinch salt

8 large eggs, beaten

¼ cup finely crumbled feta cheese

Freshly ground pepper to taste

8 teaspoons sun-dried tomato tapenade or sun-dried tomato pesto

4 whole-wheat pitas (5-inch), cut in half, warmed if desired (see Tip)

Directions

Heat oil in a large nonstick skillet over medium heat. Add spinach and salt and cook until steaming hot, stirring occasionally. Add eggs and cook, stirring the eggs as they set, until they form soft curds and are just moist, 4 to 5 minutes. Add feta and pepper and cook until set.

Spread tapenade (or pesto) inside pita pockets, 2 teaspoons per pita. Divide the egg mixture among the pitas.

Breakfast Salad with Egg & Salsa Verde Vinaigrette

Ingredients

3 tablespoons salsa verde, such as Frontera brand

1 tablespoon plus 1 tsp. extra-virgin olive oil, divided

2 tablespoons chopped cilantro, plus more for garnish

2 cups mesclun or other salad greens

8 blue corn tortilla chips, broken into large pieces

½ cup canned red kidney beans, rinsed

¼ avocado, sliced

1 large egg

Directions

Whisk salsa, 1 Tbsp. oil, and cilantro in a small bowl. Toss half the mixture with mesclun (or other greens) in a shallow dinner bowl.

Layer chips, beans, and avocado atop the salad.

Heat the remaining 1 tsp. oil in a small nonstick skillet over medium-high heat. Add egg and fry until the white is completely cooked but the yolk is still slightly runny, about 2 minutes.

Serve the egg on the salad. Drizzle with the remaining salsa vinaigrette and sprinkle with additional cilantro, if desired.

Ricotta-Berry Crepes

Ingredients

1 whole-wheat crepe

2 tablespoons low-fat ricotta cheese

¼ cup berries

1 tablespoon Honey

Directions

Spread crepe with ricotta. Top with berries. Fold up, wrap in foil and freeze for up to 1 month.

To heat and eat: Unwrap and microwave in 1-minute intervals until warmed through. Drizzle with honey, if desired.

Avocado Toast with Sprouts

Ingredients

1 cup mixed salad greens

1 teaspoon red-wine vinegar

1 teaspoon extra-virgin olive oil

Pinch of salt

Pinch of pepper

2 slices sprouted whole-wheat bread, toasted

¼ cup plain hummus

¼ cup alfalfa sprouts

¼ avocado, sliced

2 teaspoons unsalted sunflower seeds

Directions

Toss greens with vinegar, oil, salt and pepper in a medium bowl. Spread each slice of toast with 2 tablespoons hummus. Top with sprouts, avocado and the greens and sprinkle with sunflower seeds.

Salsa Egg Skillet

Ingredients

¼ cup tomatillo salsa

1 tablespoon water

1 large egg

1 tablespoon crumbled cotija cheese

1 tablespoon chopped fresh cilantro

Thinly sliced avocado, red onion and/or radishes for serving

Directions

Bring salsa and water to a simmer in a small skillet over medium heat. Make a small well in the middle and crack egg into the well. Cook, covered, until the egg is set, 3 to 5 minutes. Remove from heat and top with cheese and cilantro. Serve with avocado, onion and/or radishes, if desired.

Peanut Butter Protein Overnight Oats

Ingredients

½ cup soymilk or other plant-based milk

½ cup old-fashioned rolled oats (see Tip)

1 tablespoon pure maple syrup

1 tablespoon chia seeds

1 tablespoon powdered peanut butter

Pinch of salt

½ medium banana, sliced, or 1/2 cup berries

Directions

Stir soymilk (or other milk) sal, oats, syrup, chia, powdered peanut butter and salt together in a 2-cup mason jar. Refrigerate overnight.

Serve topped with banana or berries.

Savory Oatmeal with Tomato & Sausage

Ingredients

2 teaspoons sunflower or canola oil, divided

1 ½ ounces fully cooked sweet Italian chicken sausage (1/2 link)

1 cup low-sodium vegetable broth

½ cup old-fashioned rolled oats

⅛ teaspoon salt

½ cup grape tomatoes, halved

⅓ cup packed fresh herbs, such as parsley and/or cilantro

½ cup packed baby arugula

1 tablespoon pine nuts, toasted (see Tip)

1 large lemon wedge

Directions

Heat 1 tsp. oil in a small nonstick or cast-iron skillet over medium heat. Add sausage and cook until evenly browned, about 10 minutes.

Meanwhile, bring broth to a boil in a small saucepan over high heat. Stir in oats and salt; reduce heat to medium and cook, stirring occasionally, until the oats are tender and most of the liquid has been absorbed, about 5 minutes.

Thinly slice the sausage into coins. Stir the sausage, tomatoes, and herbs into the cooked oatmeal. Transfer to a bowl. Top with arugula and pine nuts;

drizzle with the remaining 1 tsp. oil. Serve with lemon wedge, if desired.

Spinach & Egg Scramble with Raspberries

Ingredients

1 teaspoon canola oil

1 ½ cups baby spinach (1 1/2 ounces)

2 large eggs, lightly beaten

Pinch of kosher salt

Pinch of ground pepper

1 slice whole-grain bread, toasted

½ cup fresh raspberries

Directions

Heat oil in a small nonstick skillet over medium-high heat. Add spinach and cook until wilted, stirring often, 1 to 2 minutes. Transfer the spinach to a plate. Wipe the pan clean, place over medium heat and add eggs. Cook, stirring once or twice to ensure even cooking, until just set, 1 to 2 minutes. Stir in the spinach, salt and pepper. Serve the scramble with toast and raspberries.

TASTY, YUMMY RECIPES FOR LUNCH

Herb & garlic baked cod with romesco sauce & spinach

Ingredients

2 x 140g skinless cod loin or pollock fillets

1 tbsp rapeseed oil, plus 2 tsp

1 tsp fresh thyme leaves

1 large garlic clove, finely grated

½ lemon, zested and juiced

1 large red pepper, sliced

2 leeks, well washed and thinly sliced

2 tbsp flaked almonds

1 tbsp tomato purée

¼ tsp vegetable bouillon powder

1 tsp apple cider vinegar

100g baby spinach, wilted in a pan or the microwave

Instructions

STEP 1

Heat oven to 220C/200C fan/ gas 7 and put the fish fillets in a shallow ovenproof dish so they fit quite snugly in a single layer. Mix 1 tbsp rapeseed oil with the thyme and garlic, spoon over the fish, then grate over the lemon zest. Bake for 10-12 mins until the fish is moist and flakes easily when tested.

STEP 2

Meanwhile, heat the remaining oil in a non-stick pan and fry the pepper and leeks for 5 mins until softened. Add the almonds and cook for 5 mins more. Tip in the tomato purée, 5 tbsp water, the bouillion powder and vinegar, and cook briefly to warm the mixture through.

STEP 3

Add the juice of up to half a lemon and blitz with a stick blender until it makes a thick, pesto-like sauce. Serve with the fish and the wilted spinach.

Smashed chicken with corn slaw

Ingredients

For the chicken

4 skinless chicken breast fillets

1 lime, zested and juiced

2 tbsp bio yogurt

1 tsp fresh thyme leaves

¼ tsp turmeric

2 tbsp finely chopped coriander

1 garlic clove, finely grated

1 tsp rapeseed oil

For the slaw

1 small avocado

1 lime, zested and juiced

2 tbsp bio yogurt

2 tbsp finely chopped coriander

160g corn, cut from 2 cobs

1 red pepper, deseeded and chopped

1 red onion, halved and finely sliced

320g white cabbage, finely sliced

150g new potatoes, boiled, to serve

Instructions

STEP 1

Cut the chicken breasts in half, then put them between two sheets of baking parchment and bash with a rolling pin to flatten. Mix the lime zest and juice with the yogurt, thyme, turmeric, coriander and garlic in a large bowl. Add the chicken and stir until well coated. Leave to marinate while you make the slaw.

STEP 2

Mash the avocado with the lime juice and zest, 2 tbsp yogurt and the coriander. Stir in the corn, red pepper, onion and cabbage.

STEP 3

Heat a large non-stick frying pan or griddle pan, then cook the chicken in batches for a few mins each side – they'll cook quickly as they're thin. Serve the hot chicken with the slaw and the new potatoes. If you're cooking for two, chill half the chicken and slaw for lunch another day (eat within two days).

Grilled salmon tacos with avocado salsa

Ingredients

1 tbsp smoked paprika

2 tsp ground cumin

4 skinless salmon fillets

200g natural yogurt

1 garlic clove, crushed

2 ripe avocados, stoned, peeled and diced

1 red onion, finely chopped

2 large tomatoes, deseeded and finely chopped

2 limes, juice of 1, 1 cut into wedges

small pack coriander, chopped

8 tacos shells

Instructions

STEP 1

Heat the grill to high and line a large baking tray with foil. Mix the smoked paprika and cumin in a small bowl. Rub the spices over the salmon fillets and put them on the baking tray. Pop under the grill for 8-10 mins until cooked through.

STEP 2

While the salmon cooks, combine the yogurt with the garlic and season to taste. In another bowl, combine the avocados, onion and tomatoes. Add the lime juice, season and scatter with coriander.

STEP 3

Warm the taco shells in the oven, following pack instructions. Flake the salmon and serve with the tacos, avocado salsa, yogurt and lime wedges.

Harissa vegetables with quinoa

Ingredients

1 tbsp rapeseed oil

2 red onions (160g), chopped

1 green pepper, deseeded and cubed

1 small sweet potato (200g), peeled and cut into chunks

2 large celery sticks (125g), cut into chunky slices

10g ginger, finely chopped

300ml vegetable stock made with 2 tsp vegan bouillon powder

1 tbsp harissa paste

2 tbsp tomato purée

2 dried apricots, quartered

10g coriander or parsley, chopped, plus a few extra leaves to serve

250g pack cooked red and white quinoa

4 tbsp coconut yogurt

Instructions

STEP 1

Heat the oil in a non-stick pan and fry the vegetables and ginger for 10 mins, stirring frequently, until softened and starting to colour.

STEP 2

Stir in the stock, harissa, tomato purée and apricots. Bring to the boil, cover and simmer for 15 mins. Stir in the coriander.

STEP 3

Meanwhile, heat the quinoa following pack instructions. Serve with the veg and yogurt, plus a scattering of coriander leaves.

Spaghetti with tomatoes & walnuts

Ingredients

350g wholemeal spaghetti

2 tbsp rapeseed oil

2 aubergines (about 550g), each sliced into 4 lengthways, then cut into cubes

4 large garlic cloves, finely chopped

3 tbsp tomato purée

1 tbsp balsamic vinegar

250ml vegetable stock, made with 1 tbsp bouillon powder (vegan, if needed)

330g cherry tomatoes, halved

30g pack of basil, chopped

1 tbsp capers

50g walnut pieces, lightly toasted and chopped if large

Instructions

STEP 1

Cook the spaghetti following pack instructions, then drain, reserving 150ml of the cooking water. Meanwhile, heat the oil in a large non-stick pan over a medium heat. Add the aubergine and garlic, stir well, then cover and cook for 8-10 mins, stirring a few times.

STEP 2

Mix in the tomato purée and vinegar, and cook for 2-3 mins more. Pour in the stock, then cover and cook for a further 10-15 mins until the aubergine is tender when pierced with a knife.

STEP 3

Add the cherry tomatoes and cook for a few minutes more until softened but still holding their shape. Stir in the basil, capers and walnuts, then toss through the spaghetti, adding a little of the reserved pasta water if needed to loosen. Serve half straightaway. Keep the remainder for another day.

Balsamic beef stew with veggie mash

Ingredients

1 tbsp olive or rapeseed oil

2 large onions, (325g), halved and sliced

600g diced lean stewing beef

2 garlic cloves, chopped

10g dried porcini mushrooms

2 tbsp balsamic vinegar

2 tbsp tomato purée

2 tsp vegetable bouillon powder

1 tsp English mustard powder

320g carrots, finely chopped

200g large chestnut mushrooms, quartered

few fresh thyme sprigs

4 x 80g portions broccoli, cut into florets

For the mash

750g swede, cut into chunks

500g potatoes, cut into small chunks

Instructions

STEP 1

Heat the oven to 170C/150C fan/ gas 3. Heat the oil in a heavy-based ovenproof casserole, then fry the onions for about 8 mins, stirring, until golden. Add the beef and garlic, and stir-fry over a high heat until browned all over.

STEP 2

Pour 500ml boiling water over the dried mushrooms in a bowl to briefly hydrate, then pour into the casserole with the liquid, and stir in the balsamic vinegar, tomato purée, bouillon and mustard. Pile in the carrots, chestnut mushrooms, thyme and some seasoning. Cover, then put in the oven for 3 hrs until the meat is tender. Towards the end of cooking, add a splash of water if the stew is looking dry.

STEP 3

When the stew is nearly ready, make the mash. Boil the swede and potatoes together for 12-15 mins in a pan over a medium heat. Drain well, then mash with a grating of black pepper. Steam or boil half the broccoli for 5 mins until tender. 4 Serve half the stew with the cooked broccoli. The remaining stew will keep chilled for up to three days and frozen for up a month. Defrost thoroughly before reheating. Reheat the stew and mash in the microwave and steam or boil the remaining broccoli on the night to help preserve the vitamins.

Herb & garlic baked cod with romesco sauce & spinach

Ingredients

2 x 140g skinless cod loin or pollock fillets

1 tbsp rapeseed oil, plus 2 tsp

1 tsp fresh thyme leaves

1 large garlic clove, finely grated

½ lemon, zested and juiced

1 large red pepper, sliced

2 leeks, well washed and thinly sliced

2 tbsp flaked almonds

1 tbsp tomato purée

¼ tsp vegetable bouillon powder

1 tsp apple cider vinegar

100g baby spinach, wilted in a pan or the microwave

Instructions

STEP 1

Heat oven to 220C/200C fan/ gas 7 and put the fish fillets in a shallow ovenproof dish so they fit quite snugly in a single layer. Mix 1 tbsp rapeseed oil with the thyme and garlic, spoon over the fish, then grate over the lemon zest. Bake for 10-12 mins until the fish is moist and flakes easily when tested.

STEP 2

Meanwhile, heat the remaining oil in a non-stick pan and fry the pepper and leeks for 5 mins until softened. Add the almonds and cook for 5 mins more. Tip in the tomato purée, 5 tbsp water, the bouillion powder and vinegar, and cook briefly to warm the mixture through.

STEP 3

Add the juice of up to half a lemon and blitz with a stick blender until it makes a thick, pesto-like sauce. Serve with the fish and the wilted spinach.

Noodle salad with sesame dressing

Ingredients

For the dressing

1 tbsp sesame oil

2 tsp tamari

1 lemon, juiced

1 red chilli, deseeded and finely chopped

For the salad

1 small onion, finely chopped

2 wholemeal noodle nests (about 100g)

160g sugar snap peas

4 small clementines, peeled and chopped

160g shredded carrots

large handful of coriander, chopped

50g roasted unsalted cashews

Instructions

STEP 1

Mix all the dressing Ingredients together in a large bowl, then stir in the onion. Meanwhile, cook the noodles in a pan of boiling water for 5 mins, adding the sugar snap peas halfway through the cooking time – the noodles and peas should be just tender. Drain, cool under cold running water and drain again. Snip or cut the noodles into smaller lengths to make them more manageable to eat.

STEP 2

Tip the noodles and peas into the bowl with the dressing, along with the clementines, carrots, coriander and cashews. Toss to combine, then serve in bowls or pack into rigid airtight containers to take to work.

Seared beef salad with capers & mint

Ingredients

150g new potatoes, thickly sliced

160g fine green beans, trimmed and halved

160g frozen peas

rapeseed oil, for brushing

200g lean fillet steak, trimmed of any fat

160g romaine lettuce, roughly torn into pieces

For the dressing

1 tbsp extra virgin olive oil

2 tsp cider vinegar

½ tsp English mustard powder

2 tbsp chopped mint

3 tbsp chopped basil

1 garlic clove, finely grated

1 tbsp capers

Instructions

STEP 1

Cook the potatoes in a pan of simmering water for
5 mins. Add the beans and cook 5 mins more, then

tip in the peas and cook for 2 mins until all the vegetables are just tender. Drain.

STEP 2

Meanwhile, measure all the dressing Ingredients in a large bowl and season with black pepper. Stir and crush the herbs and capers with the back of a spoon to intensify their flavours.

STEP 3

Brush a little oil over the steak and grind over some black pepper. Heat a non-stick frying pan over a high heat and cook the steak for 4 mins on one side and 2-3 mins on the other, depending on the thickness and how rare you like it. Transfer to a plate to rest while you carry on with the rest of the salad.

STEP 4

Mix the warm vegetables into the dressing until well coated, then add the lettuce and toss again. Pile onto plates. Slice the steak and turn in any dressing left in the bowl, add to the salad and serve while still warm.

Cod puttanesca with spinach & spaghetti

Ingredients

100g wholemeal spaghetti

1 large onion, sliced

1 tbsp rapeseed oil

1 red chilli, deseeded and sliced

2 garlic cloves, chopped

200g cherry tomatoes, halved

1 tsp cider vinegar

2 tsp capers

5 Kalamata olives, halved

½ tsp smoked paprika

2 skinless cod fillet or loins

160g spinach leaves

small handful chopped parsley, to serve

Instructions

STEP 1

Boil the spaghetti for 10 mins until al dente, adding the spinach for the last 2 mins. Meanwhile, fry the onion in the oil in a large non-stick frying pan with a lid until tender and turning golden. Stir in the chilli and garlic, then add the tomatoes.

STEP 2

Add the vinegar, capers, olives and paprika with a ladleful of the pasta water. Put the cod fillets on top, then cover the pan and cook for 5-7 mins until the fish just flakes. Drain the pasta and wilted spinach and pile on to plates, then top with the fish and sauce. Sprinkle over some parsley to serve.

Summer pistou

Ingredients

1 tbsp rapeseed oil

2 leeks, finely sliced

1 large courgette, finely diced

1l boiling vegetable stock (made from scratch or with reduced-salt bouillon)

400g can cannellini or haricot beans, drained

200g green beans, chopped

3 tomatoes, chopped

3 garlic cloves, finely chopped

small pack basil

40g freshly grated parmesan

Instructions

STEP 1

Heat the oil in a large pan and fry the leeks and courgette for 5 mins to soften. Pour in the stock, add three-quarters of the haricot beans with the green beans, half the tomatoes, and simmer for 5-8 mins until the vegetables are tender.

STEP 2

Meanwhile, blitz the remaining beans and tomatoes, the garlic and basil in a food processor (or in a bowl with a stick blender) until smooth, then stir in the Parmesan. Stir the sauce into the soup, cook for 1 min, then ladle half into bowls or pour into a flask for a packed lunch. Chill the remainder. Will keep for a couple of days.

Curried bean & coconut cod

Ingredients

125g brown basmati rice

200g can sweetcorn

15g ginger, peeled

2 large garlic cloves

½ tsp mustard seeds

1 tbsp garam masala

1 tsp vegetable bouillon powder

½-1 red chilli, deseeded and sliced (optional)

1 cinnamon stick

160g green beans, trimmed

160g whole cherry tomatoes

160g baby spinach

2 skinless cod loins (about 240g)

80g coconut yogurt

10g coriander, chopped, plus extra to serve

Instructions

STEP 1

Boil the rice following pack instructions. Meanwhile, tip the sweetcorn into a bowl with the ginger and garlic, and blitz with a hand blender until smooth and creamy.

STEP 2

Put the mustard seeds in a large pan and warm briefly over a low heat until they start to pop. Tip in the garam masala and sweetcorn mixture, and mix with 350ml boiling water, the bouillon, chilli (if using) and cinnamon stick. Bring to the boil, then lower the heat to medium. Add the beans and tomatoes, then cover the pan and cook for 6 mins.

STEP 3

Add the spinach and stir until beginning to wilt, then top with the fish, spoon over some sauce or gently push it under, then cover and cook 5-8 mins more until the fish is just cooked.

STEP 4

Carefully lift the fish from the pan and stir the coconut yogurt and coriander into the curry. Serve with the rice and extra coriander scattered over.

Lentil Bolognese soup

Ingredients

2 tbsp rapeseed oil

3 onions, finely chopped

3 large carrots, finely diced

3 celery sticks, finely diced

4 garlic cloves, finely chopped

500g carton passata

1 tbsp vegetable bouillon powder

125g red lentils

1 tsp smoked paprika

4 sprigs fresh thyme

125g wholemeal penne

50g finely grated vegetarian Italian-style hard cheese

Instructions

STEP 1

Heat the oil in a large non-stick pan then fry the onions for a few mins until they start to colour. Add the carrots, celery and garlic then fry for 5 more mins, stirring frequently, until the vegetables start to soften.

STEP 2

Pour in the passata, bouillon powder and the lentils with 2l boiling water. Add the smoked paprika, thyme and plenty of black pepper then bring to the boil, cover the pan and simmer for 20 mins.

STEP 3

Tip in the penne then cook for 12-15 mins more until the pasta and lentils are tender, adding a little more water if necessary. Stir through the cheese, then ladle half the soup into bowls or a wide-necked flask if you're taking it as a packed lunch. Cool the remaining soup (remove the thyme sprigs) and keep in the fridge until required. It will keep well for several days. Reheat in a pan, adding a little extra water if the soup has thickened.

TASTY, YUMMY RECIPES FOR DINNER

Air-fryer beef joint

Ingredients

1.2kg beef roasting joint

1-2 tbsp neutral-flavoured oil

1 tsp dried thyme

1 tsp onion granules

1 tsp mustard powder

Direction

STEP 1

Take the beef out of the fridge and bring it up to room temperature before cooking (20-30 mins should do it).

STEP 2

Heat the air-fryer to 220C. Rub the beef all over with the oil, then combine the thyme, onion granules and mustard powder with 1 tsp salt and 1 tsp ground black pepper in a bowl. Rub this all over the beef joint, then put the beef in the air-fryer basket and cook for 10 mins.

STEP 3

Reduce the temperature to 170C, then cook for a further 30-40 mins (30 mins for medium-rare and 40 mins for medium-well done). Transfer the meat to a board, cover loosely with foil, and leave to rest for up to 30 mins before carving and serving.

Panang chicken curry (kaeng panang gai)

Ingredients

400ml can coconut milk (don't shake to combine)

1-2 tbsp panang curry paste (see below)

200g chicken breast, thinly sliced

100g French beans, halved

2-3 tbsp fish sauce

1-2 tbsp palm sugar or brown sugar

2 makrut lime leaves, central woody stem removed, finely shredded

handful of Thai basil leaves

cooked jasmine rice, to serve

½ large red chilli, thinly sliced, to serve

For the panang curry paste (makes 225g)

4 large dried red chillies, sliced

6 large fresh red chillies, sliced

1 tsp shrimp paste (or miso paste)

4 garlic cloves, chopped

1 tbsp galangal, finely sliced

1 tbsp lemongrass, finely sliced

2 limes zested (around 1 tsp zest)

1 tsp ground white pepper

1 tsp ground coriander

1 tsp ground cumin

1 tsp ground nutmeg

2 tbsp peanuts

Direction

STEP 1

First, make the curry paste. Use a pestle and mortar to pound together the dried and fresh chillies, shrimp paste, garlic, galangal, lemongrass, lime zest, white pepper, coriander, cumin, nutmeg and peanuts, plus 1 tsp salt. You should have a rough paste. Alternatively, add all the Ingredients to a food processor along with 2-3 tbsp of coconut milk and pulse until you have a paste. Store in a lidded jar in the fridge. Will keep for up to two weeks.

STEP 2

Add 2-3 tbsp of the thick part of the coconut milk into a saucepan over a medium-high heat. When the coconut milk starts bubbling, add 1-2 tbsp of the curry paste and stir well for about 1 min, until fragrant.

STEP 3

Stir in the chicken and let it cook for about 3-4 mins until beginning to brown all over. Follow with the French beans and stir well.

STEP 4

Season with the fish sauce and sugar, then add the rest of coconut milk. Mix well, add half the makrut lime leaves and simmer for 3-5 mins until the chicken is cooked through. Taste and add more sugar or fish sauce if necessary – it should be salty and nutty, and the sweetness should come through. Add the Thai basil leaves, give it a quick mix and take off the heat. Serve with steamed jasmine rice, garnished with the sliced chilli and the rest of the makrut lime leaves.

Japchae (stir fried noodles)

Ingredients

150g dangmyun (sweet potato noodles)

1 egg

vegetable oil, for frying

100g frying steak, cut into 5mm strips

½ carrot, sliced into matchsticks

1 red pepper, thinly sliced

100g chestnut mushrooms, thinly sliced

3 spring onions, cut into 5cm lengths

sesame seeds, to garnish

For the japchae sauce

1 tbsp sesame oil

4 tbsp dark soy sauce

2 tsp caster sugar

2 tbsp toasted sesame seeds (with some extra for garnish)

1 small garlic clove, finely grated

½ tsp finely ground white pepper

For the beef marinade

1 tbsp soy sauce

2 small garlic cloves, finely grated

2 tsp caster sugar

For the spinach

200g spinach

¼ tsp salt

1 small garlic clove, finely grated

½ tsp sesame oil

2 tsp toasted sesame seeds

Direction

STEP 1

Cook the noodles following pack instructions, then drain and rinse under cold water. Mix the

Ingredients for the japchae sauce together and set aside.

STEP 2

Mix the Ingredients for the beef marinade together along with ½ tsp ground black pepper. Tip the beef into the marinade and ensure everything is thoroughly mixed. Set aside for 10 mins to marinate.

STEP 3

Place the spinach in a large heatproof bowl and cover with boiling water. Wilt for 1 min. Drain the spinach and rinse under cold water. Squeeze out any excess water. Place the drained spinach in a bowl along with the remaining spinach Ingredients and ¼ tsp salt and mix. Set to one side.

STEP 4

Crack the egg into a small bowl and stir with a fork. Place a small frying pan over a medium heat and heat the vegetable oil. Pour in the egg with a pinch of salt and move the pan around to coat it with a thin layer of the egg. Fry for 30 seconds, then flip and cook on the second side for 30 seconds to create a very thin omelette. Remove from the pan to cool, then roll into a tube shape to make it easier to slice. Slice the egg into thin strips, around 0.5cm thick. Set aside.

STEP 5

In a large frying pan, heat 1 tbsp vegetable oil over a medium heat. Using a pair of tongs, place the beef in the frying pan and fry for 1-2 mins. Remove the beef and set aside. Wipe the pan clean using kitchen paper and add 1 tsp more oil. Tip in the carrots with a pinch of salt and fry for 2 mins until slightly softened. Remove from the pan, wipe with a paper towel and add another tablespoon of oil. Fry the peppers for 2-3 mins until soft, remove from the pan, wipe clean and add another tablespoon of oil before frying the mushrooms for 6-8 mins until soft and golden.

STEP 6

Wipe out the pan and keep it on medium heat. Pour in 2 tbsp vegetable oil and when hot tip in the noodles to the pan and toss with a pair of tongs for 2 mins to heat through. Once the noodles are heated through, pour in the japchae sauce and all the other prepared Ingredients, including the spring onions. Toss the Ingredients together over a high heat for a further 2 mins, making sure everything is well combined and coated with the sauce. Serve immediately with some sesame seeds sprinkled over.

Chicken tikka

Ingredients

3 large chicken breasts, cut into chunks

75g Greek yogurt

2 tbsp ginger and garlic paste

1 tbsp madras curry powder

1 tsp ground cumin

1 tsp ground coriander

1 tsp ground turmeric

1 tsp smoked paprika

2 tsp mild chilli powder

1 tbsp lemon juice

Direction

STEP 1

Tip all of the Ingredients into a large bowl with a big pinch of salt and pepper and mix well. Cover and chill for at least a few hours, but preferably overnight.

STEP 2

Heat the grill or a barbecue to high. Thread the chicken pieces onto four metal skewers, packing the pieces in so they're all touching. Put onto a baking tray under the grill, or onto the grills of the barbecue and cook for 4-5 mins, until charred, then flip and repeat.

Brown stew chicken

Ingredients

1 whole chicken, approx 1.2kg

1 white onion, halved and thinly sliced

thumb-sized piece of ginger, grated

3 garlic cloves, crushed

3 sprigs of thyme

1 tbsp ground pimento (also known as allspice)

5 tsp caster sugar

1 tbsp soy sauce

1 red pepper, sliced

1 tbsp all-purpose seasoning

2 tbsp tomato ketchup

1 scotch bonnet pepper

2 spring onions, roughly chopped

500ml chicken stock

Direction

STEP 1

Quarter the chicken, remove the wings and separate the legs and thighs, then cut each breast into three pieces. (You can keep the carcass chilled to make stock another day.)

STEP 2

Season the chicken with the pimento, onion, all purpose seasoning, soy sauce, 1 tsp black pepper and 1½ tsp salt.

STEP 3

Add the sugar to a large pan and cook over a medium heat. Wait until the sugar starts to melt, keeping an eye on it as it starts to bubble and darken. Once it's dark brown and has gone just beyond the smell of caramel, add the chicken pieces, shaking off as much of the onion as possible.

STEP 4

Cook the chicken in batches to brown all over and remove to a pan while you cook the next batch. Once all the chicken is browned, remove from the pan and add the onion, garlic, ginger, spring onion, thyme and a pinch of salt, scraping the bowl to remove any trace of spices. Cook for 5-8 mins until the onion is soft, then return the chicken to the pan. Stir well and add the stock, scotch bonnet and tomato ketchup and top up with 100ml water. Put a lid on and cook for 20 mins. Remove the lid, add the red pepper and cook for another 20-25 mins until the sauce has thickened and the chicken has cooked through. Remove the scotch bonnet and discard, taste for seasoning and serve with rice.

Meat & potato pie

Ingredients

2 tbsp vegetable or sunflower oil

1.2kg stewing steak, cut into chunks

2 onions, sliced

2 bay leaves

2 thyme or rosemary sprigs

750ml beef stock

750g Maris Piper potatoes, halved, quartered if large

1-2 tsp cornflour

320g pack ready-rolled shortcrust pastry, or 500g block shortcrust pastry

plain flour, for dusting

1 egg, beaten

Direction

STEP 1

Heat the oil in a large lidded pan over a medium heat and brown the meat well all over (you may need to do this in batches). This will take 20-25 mins. Remove to a plate and set aside.

STEP 2

Fry the onions in the pan for 3-4 mins until starting to brown, then return the meat to the pan and add the bay leaves and thyme or rosemary. Pour in the stock and bring to a simmer. Cook for 1 hr 30 mins-2 hrs, checking every 30 mins until the meat is tender.

STEP 3

Tip in the potatoes and cook for 10-12 mins more until the potatoes are just cooked through. Remove 2 tbsp liquid from the pan and combine with the cornflour to make a paste, then pour this back into the mixture, stir and simmer until thickened. Remove from the heat and tip the filling into a large ovenproof dish.

STEP 4

Heat the oven to 200C/180C fan/gas 6. Roll the pastry out on a lightly floured surface into a rectangle the thickness of a 50p piece large enough to cover the dish. Lay the pastry rectangle over the dish and crimp it around the rim of the dish to seal, trimming any excess. Cut two holes in the top of the pastry to allow any steam to escape, then brush over the beaten egg. Bake for 20-30 mins until the pastry is golden. Leave to rest for a few minutes, then serve hot.

Vegetarian enchiladas

Ingredients

1 tsp olive oil

2 onions, chopped

280g carrots, grated

2-3 tsp chilli powder (mild or hot, according to your taste)

2 x 400g cans chopped tomatoes

2 x 400g cans pulses in water, drained (we used mixed beans and lentils)

6 small wholemeal tortillas

200g low-fat natural yogurt

50g extra-mature cheddar cheese (or veg alternative), finely grated

Direction

STEP 1

Heat the oil in a large frying pan. Cook the onions and carrots for 5-8 mins until soft – add a splash of water if they start to stick. Sprinkle in the chilli powder and cook for 1 min more. Pour in the tomatoes and pulses and bring to the boil. Turn down the heat and simmer for 5-10 mins, stirring occasionally, until thickened. Remove from the heat and season well.

STEP 2

Heat grill to high. Spread a spoonful of the bean chilli over a large ovenproof dish. Lay each tortilla onto a board, fill with a few tbsp of chilli mixture, fold over the ends and roll up to seal. Place them into the ovenproof dish. Spoon the remaining chilli on top.

STEP 3

Mix the yogurt and grated cheese together with some seasoning, and spoon over the enchiladas. Grill for a few mins until the top is golden and bubbling. Serve with a green salad.

Chickpea & coriander burgers

Ingredients

400g can chickpeas, drained

zest 1 lemon, plus juice ½

1 tsp ground cumin

small bunch coriander, chopped

1 egg

100g fresh breadcrumbs

1 medium red onion, ½ diced, ½ sliced

1 tbsp olive oil

4 small wholemeal buns

1 large tomato, sliced, ½ cucumber, sliced and chilli sauce, to serve

Direction

STEP 1

In a food processor, whizz the chickpeas, lemon zest, lemon juice, cumin, half the coriander, the egg and some seasoning. Scrape into a bowl and mix with 80g of the breadcrumbs and the diced onions. Form 4 burgers, press remaining breadcrumbs onto both sides and chill for at least 10 mins.

STEP 2

Heat the oil in a frying pan until hot. Fry the burgers for 4 mins each side, keeping the heat on medium so they don't burn. To serve, slice each bun and fill with a slice of tomato, a burger, a few red onion slices, some cucumber slices, a dollop of chilli sauce and the remaining coriander.

Giant couscous salad with charred veg & tangy pesto

Ingredients

2-3 raw beetroot (320g), peeled and chopped

3 red onions (320g), cut into wedges

2 green or orange peppers, deseeded and cubed

1 tbsp olive oil

320g cherry tomatoes

200g wholewheat giant couscous

For the pesto

7g fresh coriander, roughly chopped

15g flat-leaf parsley, roughly chopped

1 garlic clove

1 green chilli, deseeded

½ tsp cumin

1 tbsp apple cider vinegar

1 tbsp olive oil

40g pine nuts, lightly toasted

Direction

STEP 1

Heat the oven to 200C/180C fan/gas 6. In a bowl, toss the beetroot, onions and peppers together with the oil, then spread out on a large roasting tray lined with baking paper and roast for 35 mins. Scatter over the cherry tomatoes, then return to the oven for 10 mins more until the tomatoes have softened and the vegetables are tender.

STEP 2

Meanwhile, cook the couscous following pack instructions, then rinse and drain. To make the pesto, put the coriander and half the parsley in a bowl with the garlic, chilli, cumin, vinegar, oil and 25g of the pine nuts. Add 2 tbsp water, then blitz with a hand blender until smooth or use a small food processor.

STEP 3

Toss the roasted veg and chopped parsley through the couscous and pile on the pesto, then scatter with the remaining pine nuts

Courgette curry with lemon rice

Ingredients

For the curry

1 tbsp olive oil

2 tbsp ginger, very finely chopped

1½ tsp cumin seeds

1-2 red chillies, deseeded and finely chopped

6 garlic cloves, crushed

450g baby potatoes, thickly sliced

2 tsp ground coriander

1 tsp ground turmeric

4 large vine tomatoes, roughly chopped

1 tbsp tomato purée

200ml stock, made with 1 tsp vegetable bouillon powder

1 cinnamon stick

500g medium-sized courgettes, thickly sliced

15g chopped fresh coriander

For the lemon rice

1 tbsp olive oil

½-1 tsp brown mustard seeds (optional)

240g brown basmati rice

½-1 tsp turmeric

12 curry leaves (optional)

400g can chickpeas, drained

2 tbsp lemon juice

Direction

STEP 1

Heat the oil in a large frying pan and fry the ginger for 3 mins. Stir in the cumin seeds, chillies and garlic and cook briefly, then add the potatoes, ground coriander and turmeric, and stir well. Tip in the tomatoes, tomato purée and stock, then add the cinnamon, cover, and leave to simmer for 5 mins.

STEP 2

Stir in the courgettes, then cover and cook for 10-12 mins until the courgettes are tender rather than soft. Stir in the fresh coriander.

STEP 3

Meanwhile, heat the oil in a pan and stir in the mustard seeds, if using, and cook until you hear them pop. Stir in the rice, turmeric and curry leaves, if using, then pour in 1 litre boiling water. Simmer, covered, for 15 mins, then add the chickpeas and lemon juice, cover once again, and cook for 10 mins more until the water has been absorbed and the rice is tender.

Turkey chilli

Ingredients

1 tbsp rapeseed oil

500g turkey thigh mince (7% fat)

2 large garlic cloves, finely grated

1 chilli, deseeded and chopped

½ tsp dried oregano

2 tsp ground coriander

1 tsp ground cumin

1 tbsp smoked paprika

500g carton passata

2 x 400g cans red kidney beans drained (liquid reserved)

2 tsp vegetable bouillon powder

2 red peppers, deseeded and diced

4 small sweet potatoes (about 140g each)

2 avocados

1 lime, juiced

Direction

STEP 1

Heat the oil in a large pan over a medium heat, then tip in the mince and break it up using a wooden spoon. Stir in the garlic and chilli, and cook for 10 mins until the mince is cooked through. Add the herbs and spices, and cook for a minute more.

STEP 2

Pour in the passata, the reserved liquid from the beans, the bouillon powder and peppers. Cover and cook for 15-20 mins until slightly thickened. Tip in the beans and cook for 3-5 mins more.

STEP 3

Meanwhile, prick two of the sweet potatoes all over using a fork, then microwave on high for 7-10 mins until tender. Mash one of the avocados with half the lime juice in a small bowl.

STEP 4

To serve, halve the potatoes and spoon over half the chilli, then finish with the mashed avocado. Chill the remainder for another day. The chilli will keep covered and chilled for four days or frozen for three months. Reheat in a microwave or pan over low heat until piping hot. Serve with the remaining sweet potatoes and mashed avocado and lime juice, as described above.

Turmeric chicken with butter bean hummus & roasted peppers

Ingredients

1 large red pepper, halved and deseeded

1 tsp vegetable oil

160g long-stem broccoli

handful of mint leaves, to serve

For the chicken and marinade

2 large skinless chicken breast fillets (about 125g each)

120g natural yogurt

3 tbsp finely grated turmeric

½ tsp cumin seeds

½ tsp ground coriander

1 garlic clove, finely grated

1 tbsp lemon juice

1 tsp honey

1 tsp extra virgin olive oil

For the butter bean hummus

400g can butter beans, drained, liquid reserved

1 tbsp lemon zest, plus 1 tbsp lemon juice

1 tbsp extra virgin olive oil, plus a drizzle

1 garlic clove, roughly chopped

½ tsp cumin seeds

½ tsp ground coriander

Direction

STEP 1

Heat the oven to 220C/200C fan/gas 7. Line a baking sheet with foil. Make a few small cuts around the edges of the pepper halves using a sharp knife, then flatten them as much as you can with your palm. Rub with the veg oil and roast on the lined baking sheet for 10 mins.

STEP 2

Meanwhile, cut the chicken breasts in half lengthways at an angle so you end up with four thin fillets. Mix the yogurt, turmeric, cumin seeds, ground coriander, garlic, lemon juice, honey and olive oil with some black pepper and 1 tsp salt in a bowl. Add the chicken and turn to coat in the marinade. When the peppers have had 10 mins, turn them over, add the chicken fillets to the sheet, spacing them apart slightly, and spoon any remaining marinade over them. Roast for 20 mins, turning the chicken fillets halfway, until cooked through.

STEP 3

For the hummus, use a hand blender to blitz together the beans, lemon zest and juice, olive oil, garlic, cumin seeds and coriander with 6 tbsp liquid from the can, ¾ tsp salt and plenty of black pepper. It should be completely smooth.

STEP 4

When the chicken has been cooking for 10 mins, steam the broccoli for 6 mins until tender. Spoon the hummus over two plates, then top with the roasted peppers and chicken. Scatter with the mint, drizzle with olive oil and serve with the broccoli on the side.

Spiced fried rice with sausage

Ingredients

275g long-grain rice

2 eggs

4 tbsp garlic-infused oil

1 red pepper, cut into 1cm cubes

2 carrots, cut into 1cm cubes

6 cooked gluten-free pork sausages, sliced on the diagonal

3 tbsp gluten-free soy sauce

2 tbsp curry powder

1 tsp ground turmeric

2 tsp caster sugar

100g frozen peas

1 bunch of spring onions, greens finely chopped (use the white parts in another recipe)

Direction

STEP 1

Cook the rice following pack instructions, then drain if needed and leave to cool completely. Cover and chill overnight.

STEP 2

Crack the eggs into a small bowl, add a pinch of salt and beat briefly using a fork. Heat the oil in a large wok over a medium-high heat and, once hot, stir-fry the red pepper and carrots until lightly browned. Add the cooked sausage and beaten egg, cook without stirring for 30 seconds, then break the egg up into chunks using a wooden spoon.

STEP 3

Stir in the cooked rice, breaking it up as you do, then add the soy sauce, curry powder, turmeric and caster sugar, and stir again to coat the rice. Tip in the frozen peas and stir-fry for 5 mins more, or until the rice has crisped up in places. Serve the fried rice topped with the spring onion greens.

Butternut squash, sausage, spinach & mushroom pasta bake

Ingredients

1 butternut squash (about 900g), peeled, deseeded and cut into 2-3cm cubes

2 tbsp olive oil, plus extra for the dish

6 sausages (about 400g)

50g unsalted butter

sage (about 10 leaves)

50g plain flour

500ml whole milk, plus extra for topping up, if needed

nutmeg, grated

40g grated parmesan, plus extra to serve

1 tbsp Dijon mustard

300g fusilli

70g mushrooms, sliced

1 garlic clove, crushed

100g kale, chard or spinach, chopped

Direction

STEP 1

Heat the oven to 200C/180 fan/gas 6. Put the squash in a roasting tin, toss with 1 tbsp olive oil and season. Cut each sausage into three, arrange them around the squash and roast for 35-40 mins, turning halfway, until the squash is tender and the sausages are caramelised.

STEP 2

Meanwhile, melt the butter in a saucepan over a medium heat, until bubbling. Add the sage and allow to sizzle for a few minutes, or until crisp. Remove with a slotted spoon and set aside on a plate lined with kitchen paper. By this point, the butter should have browned. Stir in the flour and cook for a few seconds, then gradually pour in the milk, whisking continuously, until you have a smooth sauce – this should take around 7-10 mins. Add the nutmeg, season, stir in the parmesan until melted, then stir in the mustard.

STEP 3

Oil a medium-sized baking dish. Cook the pasta following pack instructions until al dente, then drain and run under cold water. Heat the remaining 1 tbsp oil in a pan over a medium heat and fry the mushrooms with a pinch of salt for a few minutes, until softened and caramelised. Add the garlic, then the greens, stirring until wilted, then add to the white sauce along with the squash, pasta and half the fried sage, adding up to 50ml milk or water if it's too thick.

STEP 4

Pour into the baking dish, then add the sausages. Scatter over the remaining sage and some extra grated parmesan. Roast for 25-30 mins, until golden and bubbling. Allow to settle for 10 mins before serving.

TASTY, YUMMY RECIPES FOR SNACK OPTIONS

Tteokbokki (spicy rice cakes)

Ingredients

500g garaetteok (cylindrical rice cakes)

500ml vegetable stock or water

2½ tbsp gochujang (Korean red pepper paste)

2 tbsp soy sauce

3½ tbsp sugar

1 tbsp corn syrup

200g eomuk (Korean fish cakes), roughly cut

3 spring onions, cut into thirds

Directions

STEP 1

If using refrigerated rice cakes, soak in warm water for 15 mins. Place a large frying pan over high heat and pour in the stock (or water). Bring to a boil, then add the gochujang, soy sauce, sugar and corn syrup. Stir and reduce to a medium heat.

STEP 2

Tip the rice cakes and fish cakes into the pan of sauce. Simmer for 10 mins until the rice cakes are soft and the sauce has thickened and clings to the rice cakes. Stir in the spring onions and serve immediately.

Mozzarella, pepper & aubergine calzone

Ingredients

400g strong wholewheat bread flour, plus extra for dusting

⅛ tsp salt (optional)

7g sachet fast-action dried yeast

2 tsp rapeseed oil, plus extra for the baking sheet

For the filling

2 tsp rapeseed oil

1 red and 1 yellow pepper, deseeded and cut into small chunks

1 large aubergine, halved lengthways and thinly sliced

2 large garlic cloves, finely chopped

1 tbsp tomato purée

1 tbsp balsamic vinegar

small bunch basil, roughly torn

8 pitted Kalamata olives, halved

125g ball mozzarella (drained weight), quartered

milk or beaten egg, for brushing

Directions

STEP 1

Put the flour, salt (if using), yeast, oil and 300ml lukewarm water in a bowl and mix until soft. Knead into a ball (try not to add any extra flour) – it will be sticky but the flour will absorb some moisture.

Return to the bowl, cover and leave somewhere warm.

STEP 2

Meanwhile, make the filling. Heat the oil in a large non-stick pan, then stir-fry the peppers for about 1 min until they start to soften. Add the aubergine and garlic and continue to cook over a medium heat for 8-10 mins, gently pressing the veg with a wooden spoon until it breaks down a little. If it doesn't, fry, covered, for a few extra mins.

STEP 3

Stir in the tomato purée, vinegar and 2 tbsp water. When the veg is soft, remove the pan from the heat and stir through the basil.

STEP 4

Heat the oven to 220C/200C fan/gas 7. Quarter the risen dough and roll each piece out to a 20cm circle on a lightly floured surface. Spoon a quarter of the filling over one side, scatter over a quarter of the olives, top with a quarter of the cheese, and brush the edges with the milk or beaten egg. Fold the dough over the filling and pinch the edges together at the side, a bit like making a Cornish pasty. Lift onto a lightly oiled baking sheet and brush with more milk or beaten egg. Repeat with the remaining dough and filling to make four calzones, then bake for 15-20 mins until golden. Leave to cool slightly and serve at room temperature.

Crispy roasted chickpeas

Ingredients

1 x 400g can chickpeas, drained

1tsp rapeseed oil

2tsp smoked paprika

2tsp ground cumin

2tsp ground coriander

½tsp cayenne pepper

Directions

STEP 1

Heat oven to 200C/180C fan/gas 4. Tip the chickpeas into a bowl and toss with the rapeseed oil, smoked paprika, cumin and coriander along with a big pinch of salt. Toss well until the chickpeas are well coated, then tip out onto a baking tray and bake for 35 mins, moving them round the tray halfway through so they dry out evenly and are crunchy. Leave to cool, then store in an airtight container.

Healthy tuna lettuce wraps

Ingredients

2 drops rapeseed oil, for brushing

2 x 140g fresh tuna fillets, defrosted

1 ripe avocado

½ tsp English mustard powder

1 tsp cider vinegar

1 tbsp capers

8 romaine lettuce leaves

16 cherry tomatoes, preferably on the vine, halved

Directions

STEP 1

Brush the tuna with a little oil. Heat a non-stick pan, add the tuna and cook for 1 min each side, or a min or so longer for a thicker fillet. Transfer to a plate to rest.

STEP 2

Halve and stone the avocado and scoop the flesh into a small bowl. Add the mustard powder and vinegar, then mash well so that the mixture is smooth like mayonnaise. Stir in the capers. Spoon into two small dishes and put on serving plates with the lettuce leaves, and tomatoes.

STEP 3

Slice the tuna (it should be slightly pink inside) and arrange on the plates. Spoon some 'mayo' on the lettuce leaves and top with tuna and cherry tomatoes and a few extra capers. To eat, roll up into little wraps.

Fruit & nut breakfast bowl

Ingredients

6 tbsp porridge oats

2 oranges

just under ½ x 200ml tub 0% fat Greek-style yogurt

60g pot raisins, nuts, goji berries and seeds

Directions

STEP 1

Put the oats in a non-stick pan with 400ml water and cook over the heat, stirring occasionally for about 4 mins until thickened.

STEP 2

Meanwhile, cut the peel and pith from the oranges then slice them in half, cutting down either side, as closely as you can, to where the stalk would be as this will remove quite a tough section of the membrane. Now just chop the oranges.

STEP 3

Pour the porridge into bowls, spoon on the yogurt then pile on the oranges and the fruit, nut and seed mixture.

Quinoa, peach & ginger bircher

Ingredients

200g quinoa

200g porridge oats

4 tsp finely grated ginger

225ml milk, plus a little extra if required

1 tbsp vanilla extract

6 x 120ml pots bio yogurt

6 ripe peaches

Directions

STEP 1

Boil the quinoa in plenty of cold water for about 18 mins until the grains burst. Tip into a sieve and rinse under under cold water. Meanwhile, tip the oats into a large bowl with the ginger. Pour over 400ml boiling water and stir well. The mixture will become quite thick, but this process does stop the slightly starchy taste that some birchers made with cold water have. Stir in 225ml milk, the vanilla and 3 pots of yogurt, then fold through the quinoa. Cover and chill overnight.

STEP 2

The next day, add a little more milk to get the consistency you want, then spoon into six bowls. Top two with a ½ pot yogurt each and 2 stoned and chopped peaches, then mix together.

Deconstructed guacamole

Ingredients

2 tomatoes, finely chopped

4 tsp finely chopped red onion

2 tsp finely chopped coriander

1 small avocado, halved and stoned

pinch of chilli powder, hot or mild, to taste

2 small lime wedges, to serve

Directions

STEP 1

Mix the tomatoes, onion and coriander in a bowl. Spoon onto the avocado halves, sprinkle with a little chilli powder, then serve with a lime wedge each for squeezing over.

Tuna Niçoise protein pot

Ingredients

1 large egg

80g green beans

1 tomato, amber or red, quartered

120g can tuna in spring water

1½ -2 tbsp French dressing

Directions

STEP 1

Boil the egg for 8-10 mins depending on if you want a soft or hard yolk, then at the same time steam the green beans for 6 mins above the pan until tender. Cool the egg and beans under running water then carefully shell and quarter the egg. Leave to cool.

STEP 2

Tip the beans into a large packed lunch pot. Top with the tomato, tuna and quartered egg and spoon on the French dressing. Seal until ready to eat

Rainbow rice

Ingredients

100g basmati rice, long grain rice or brown rice

1small red pepper, deseeded and finely chopped

½ cucumber, deseeded and finely chopped

1large carrot, grated

6 dried apricots, chopped

2 tbsp toasted pumpkin seed or sunflower seeds

2 tbsp olive oil

½ orange, juice only

Directions

STEP 1

Cook the rice as per pack instructions. Drain, rinse and drain again. Mix with the red pepper, cucumber, grated carrot, dried apricots and toasted pumpkin seeds. Drizzle over olive oil and the orange juice.

Avocado & strawberry ices

Ingredients

200g ripe strawberries, hulled and chopped

1 avocado, stoned, peeled and roughly chopped

2 tsp balsamic vinegar

½ tsp vanilla extract

1-2 tsp maple syrup (optional)

Directions

STEP 1

Put the strawberries (save four pieces for the top), avocado, vinegar and vanilla in a bowl and blitz using a hand blender (or in a food processor) until as smooth as you can get it. Have a taste and only add the maple syrup if the strawberries are not sweet enough.

STEP 2

Pour into containers, add a strawberry to each, cover with cling film and freeze. Allow the pots to soften for 5-10 mins before eating.

Masala omelette muffins

Ingredients

olive oil, for greasing

2 medium courgettes, coarsely grated

6 large eggs

2 large or 4 small garlic cloves, finely grated

1 red chilli, deseeded and finely chopped

1 tsp chilli powder

1 tsp ground cumin

1 tsp ground coriander

handful fresh coriander, chopped

125g frozen peas

40g feta

Directions

STEP 1

Heat oven to 220C/200C fan/ gas 7 and lightly oil four 200ml ramekins. Grate the courgettes and squeeze really well, removing as much liquid as possible. Put all the Ingredients except the feta in a large jug and mix really well.

STEP 2

Pour into the ramekins, scatter with the feta and bake on a baking sheet for 20-25 mins until risen and set. You can serve the muffins hot or cold with salad, slaw or cooked vegetables.

Bean & feta spread with Greek salad salsa & oatcakes

Ingredients

400g can butter beans, drained

1 lemon, ½ juiced, ½ cut into 4 wedges

2 tbsp ricotta or bio yogurt

85g feta, crumbled

1 garlic clove

12 oatcakes

For the salsa

4 tomatoes, chopped

1 medium cucumber, finely diced

1 small red onion, finely chopped

12 pitted Kalamata olives, chopped

a few chopped mint leaves (optional)

Directions

STEP 1

Tip the beans, lemon juice, ricotta, 50g feta and the garlic into a bowl and blitz with a hand blender or in a food processor to make a paste. Stir in the remaining feta and spoon the mixture into four small pots.

STEP 2

To make the salsa, stir all the Ingredients together with the mint (if using) and divide into four more pots, topping with a lemon wedge. These will keep, chilled in an airtight container, for two-three days. To eat, spread the oatcakes with the bean mixture, squeeze the lemon wedges over the salads and pile generously onto the oatcakes.

Chia & oat breakfast scones with yogurt and berries

Ingredients

2 tsp cold pressed rapeseed oil, plus a little for the ramekins

50ml milk

1 tbsp lemon juice

2 tsp vanilla extract

160g plain wholemeal spelt flour

2 tbsp chia seeds

25g oats

2 tsp baking powder

2 x 120g pots bio Greek yogurt

400g strawberries, hulled and sliced

Directions

STEP 1

Heat oven to 200C/180C fan/gas 6 and line the base of 4 x 185ml ramekins with a disc of baking parchment and oil the sides with the rapeseed oil.

Measure the milk in a jug and make up to 300ml with water. Stir in the lemon juice, vanilla and the 2 tsp oil. Mix the flour, seeds and oats then blitz in a food processor to make the mix as fine as you can. Stir in the baking powder.

STEP 2

Pour in the liquid, then stir in with the blade of a knife until you have a very wet batter like dough. Spoon evenly into the ramekins then bake on a baking sheet for 20 mins until risen – they don't have to be golden but should feel firm. Cool for a few mins then run a knife round the inside of the ramekins to loosen the scones then carefully ease out.

STEP 3

The scones can be eaten immediately or cooled and stored for later.

Chapter 5: FINAL THOUGHTS

In summary, while tweaking your diet might offer some relief for amyloidosis symptoms, it's not a substitute for proper medical care or a cure. Opting for a balanced diet loaded with anti-inflammatory foods, steering clear of excessive sugars, and moderating protein intake could potentially ease the burden of the condition. Still, it's crucial to consult with healthcare pros or dietitians to tailor these changes to your specific needs. And let's not forget, ongoing research is key. We're still unraveling the intricate ties between what we eat and how it affects amyloidosis, which could lead to more targeted dietary strategies down the road.